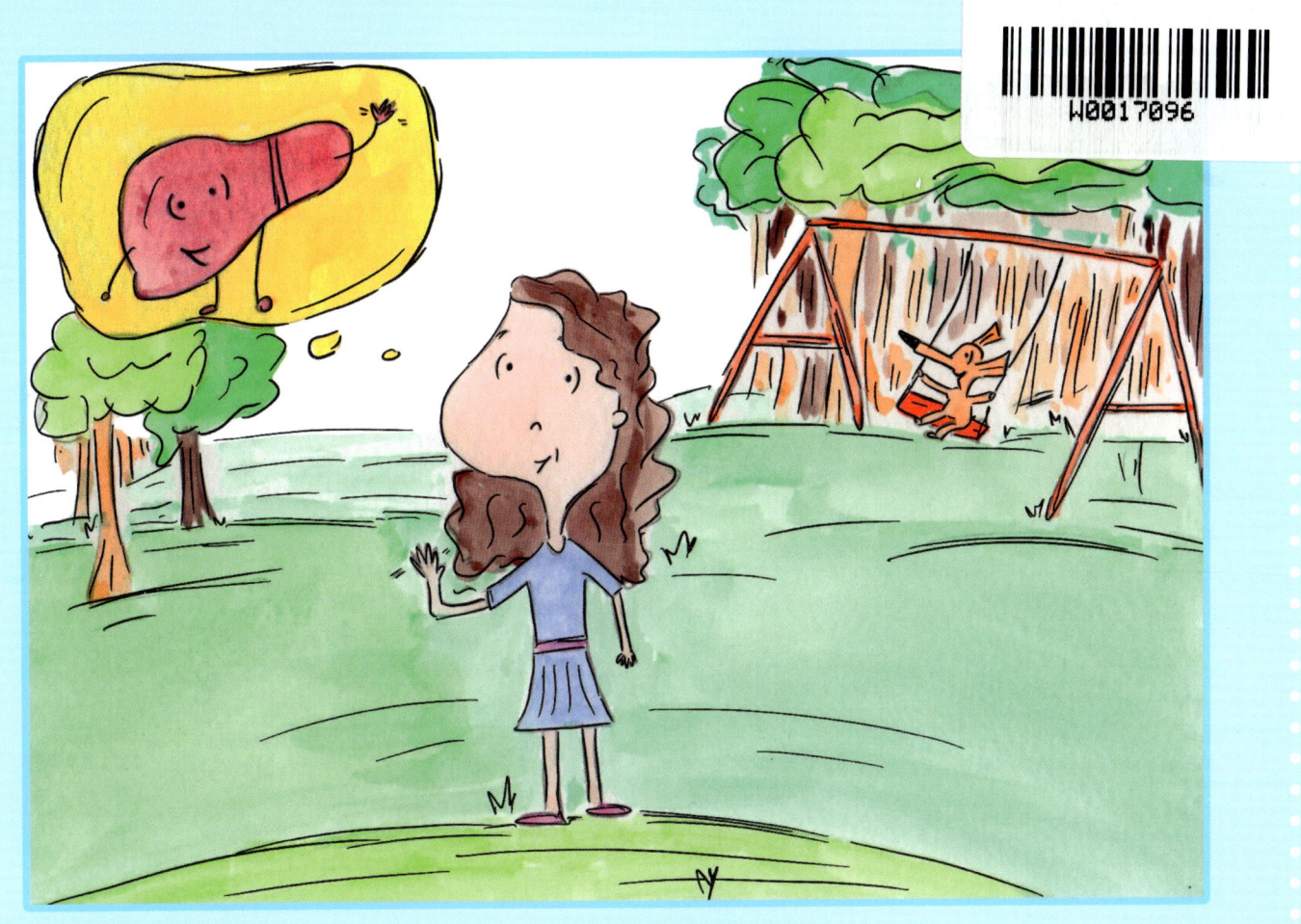

Hello there! I hear you are on your way to a liver transplant! So, what happens when your new liver is found? Good question. I'm here to tell you all about it!

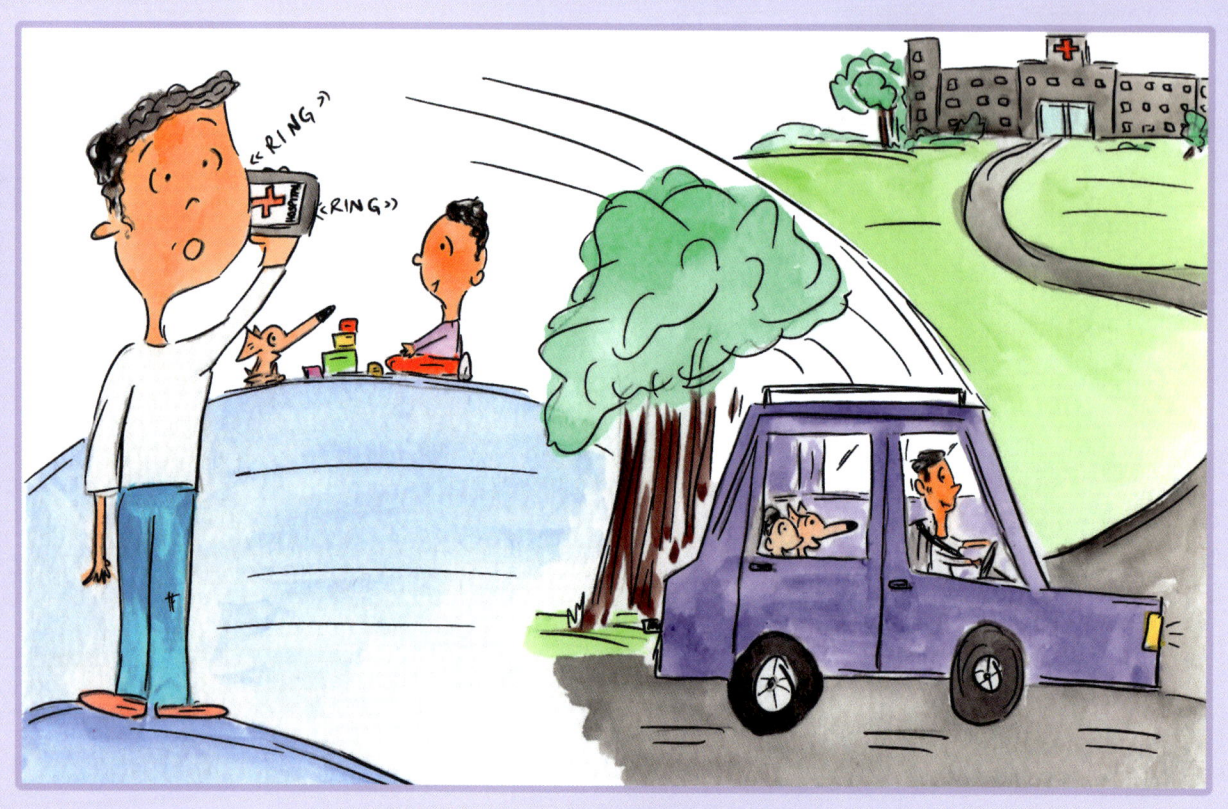

Step 1. The phone call

When a new liver is found and is the right match to you, you will get a phone call. RING, RING. Time to head to the hospital! Don't let your parents speed! We want you to get there safe and sound. And don't worry – you will be told exactly when to stop eating and drinking.

(If your new liver is from a living donor, you will know the day and time of surgery well in advance. So, no surprise phone call!)

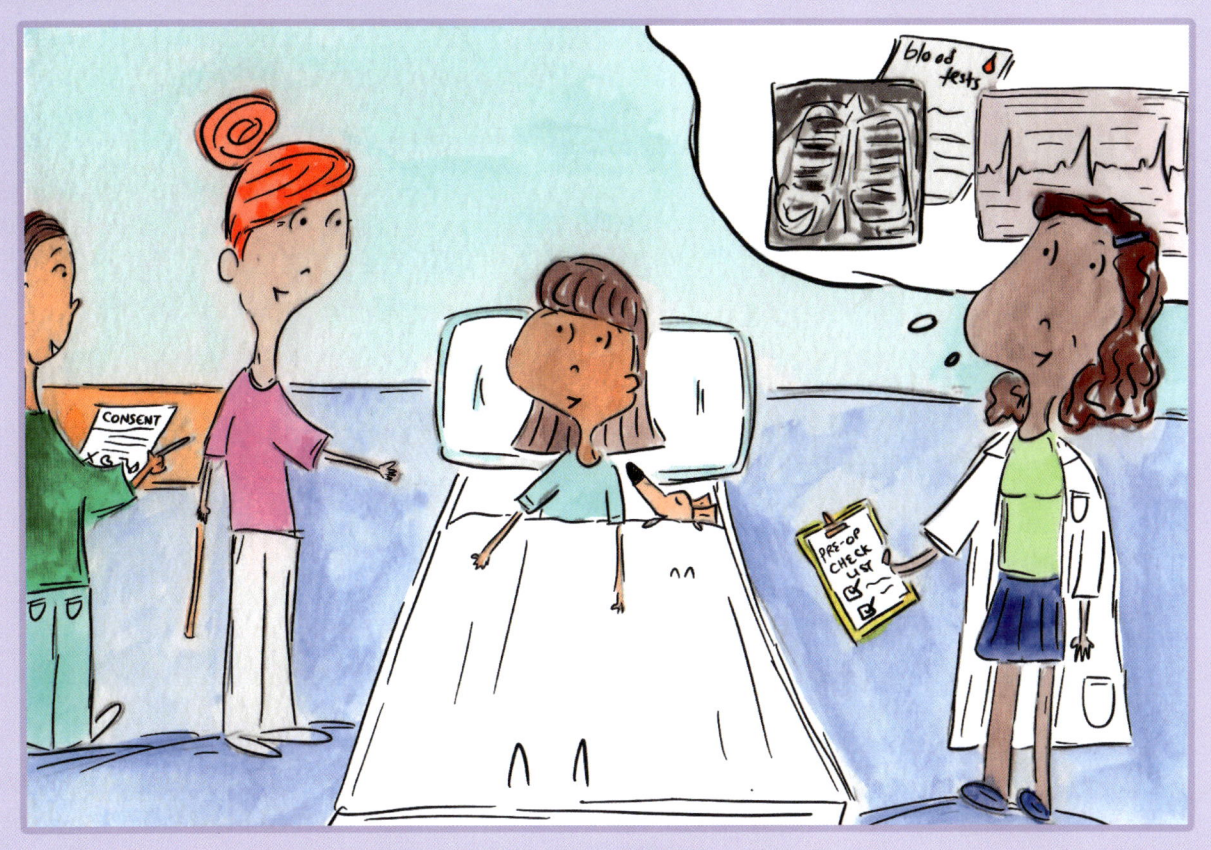

Step 2. Checklist time

Once at the hospital, you will get checked up and down. Lab blood tests will be drawn. An **x-ray** of your chest will be taken. Your heart will be looked at using an **EKG** (stickers are put on your chest to look at your heart – this doesn't hurt!). And your doctors will come see you. Your parents will sign permission slip forms for the transplant surgery. These are called **consents**.

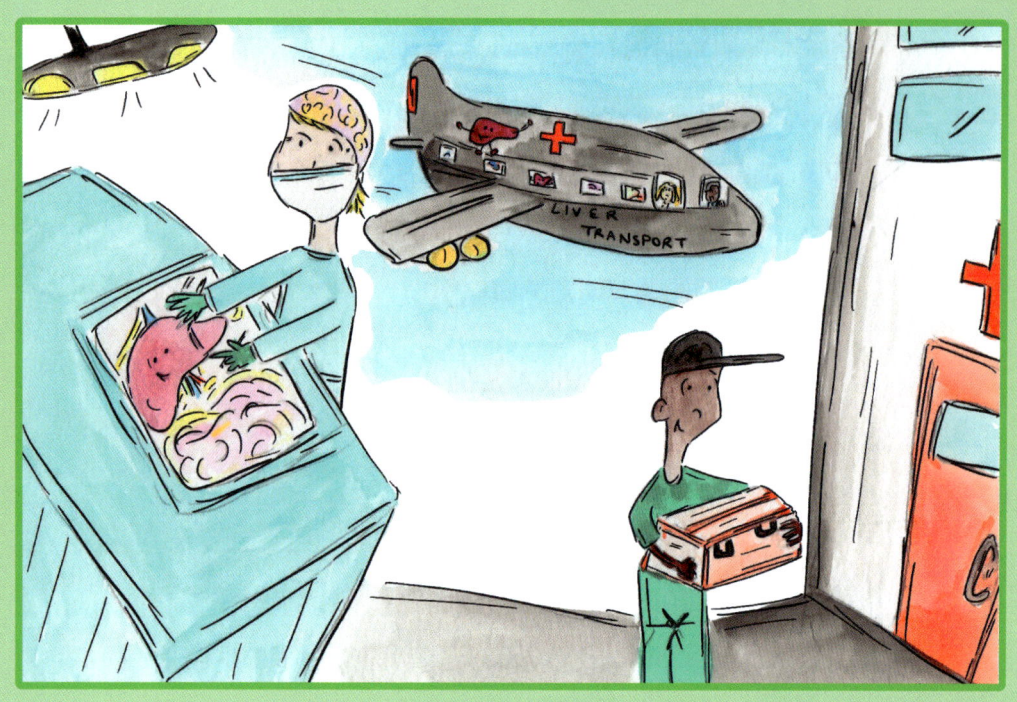

Step 3A. The donor hepatectomy – deceased cadaveric

This is the first surgery. You're not a part of this one. It's when your team goes and gets your new liver. If it's from a deceased (cadaveric) liver – remember the green truck* – your team will go get it to bring it back for you. Sometimes when they see the liver, they realize it's not perfect. And your surgery may be canceled. Because we only want a perfect liver for you! If it is perfect, they'll bring the liver back, and we'll move on to the second surgery.

*the green truck from our book *Liver Transplantation Part One: The Basics,* represents a person who has sadly died, and donated their liver to people in need.

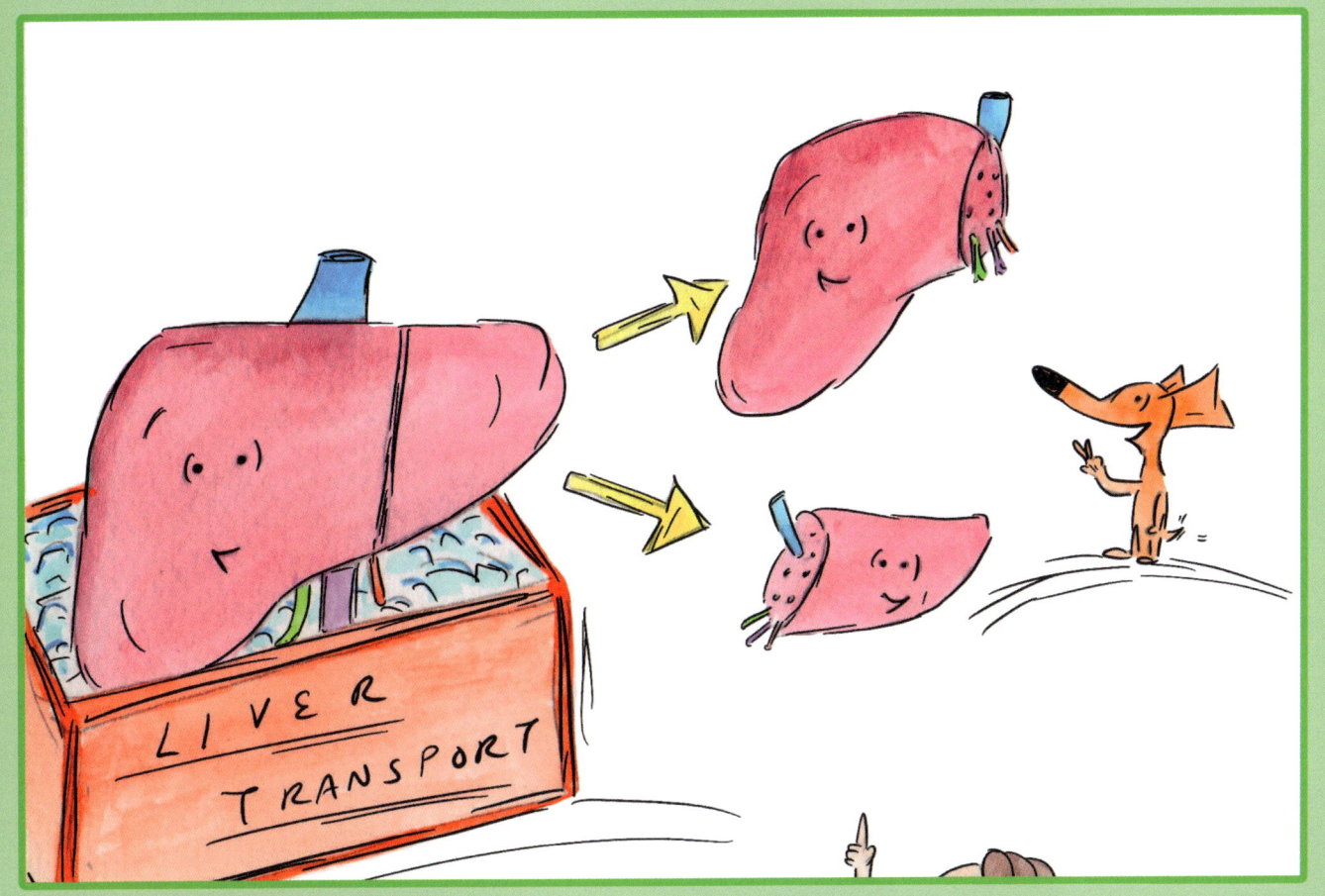

Step 3B. The donor hepatectomy – deceased cadaveric split

Sometimes the new liver we choose for you is too big for your body. So, we cut it in two pieces. This is called a **SPLIT** liver. Remember livers **regenerate** (or regrow) so you really only need a piece of liver. It grows to a normal size within weeks.

How crazy is that?!

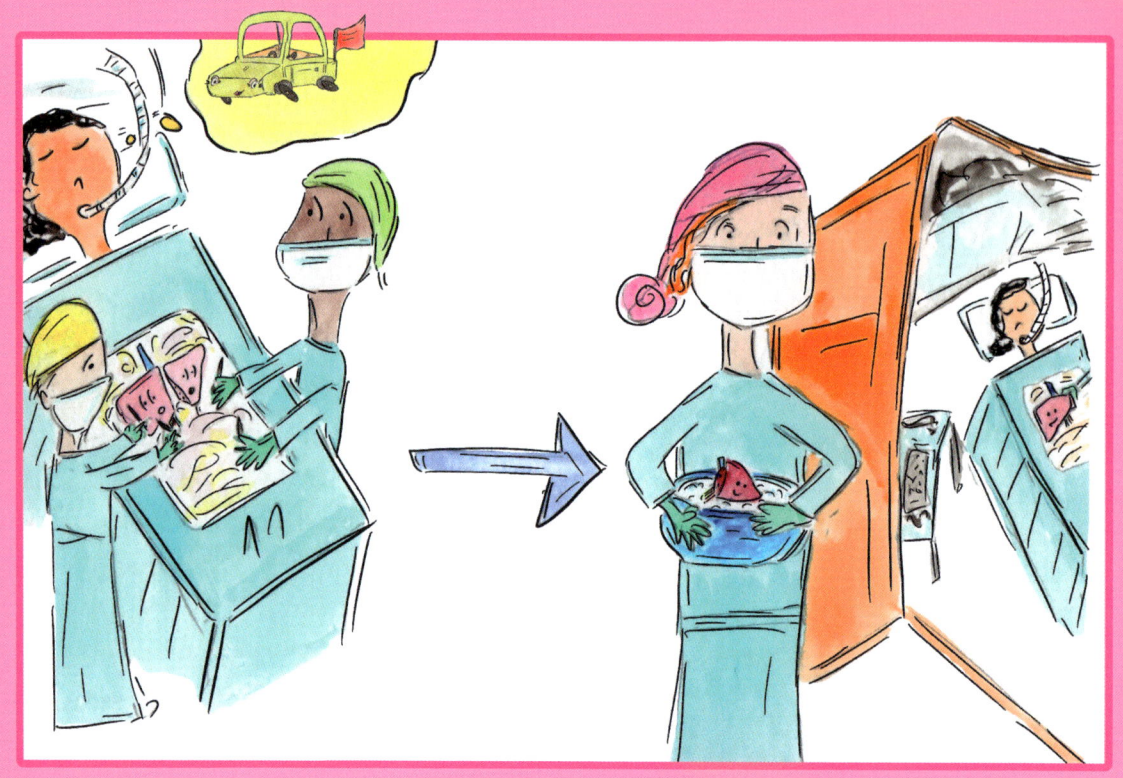

Step 3C. The donor hepatectomy – living donor

Sometimes your new liver is a gift from someone alive (like your mom or dad!). You get a piece of their liver to replace your sick liver – remember the yellow beetle*! In this case, your team will start taking out the piece of liver from your "**living donor**". Sometimes they do this **robotically** – how cool is that?! As they operate, you'll be getting ready for your surgery!

*the yellow beetle from our book Liver Transplantation Part One: The Basics, represents a living person who gifts you a piece of their liver.

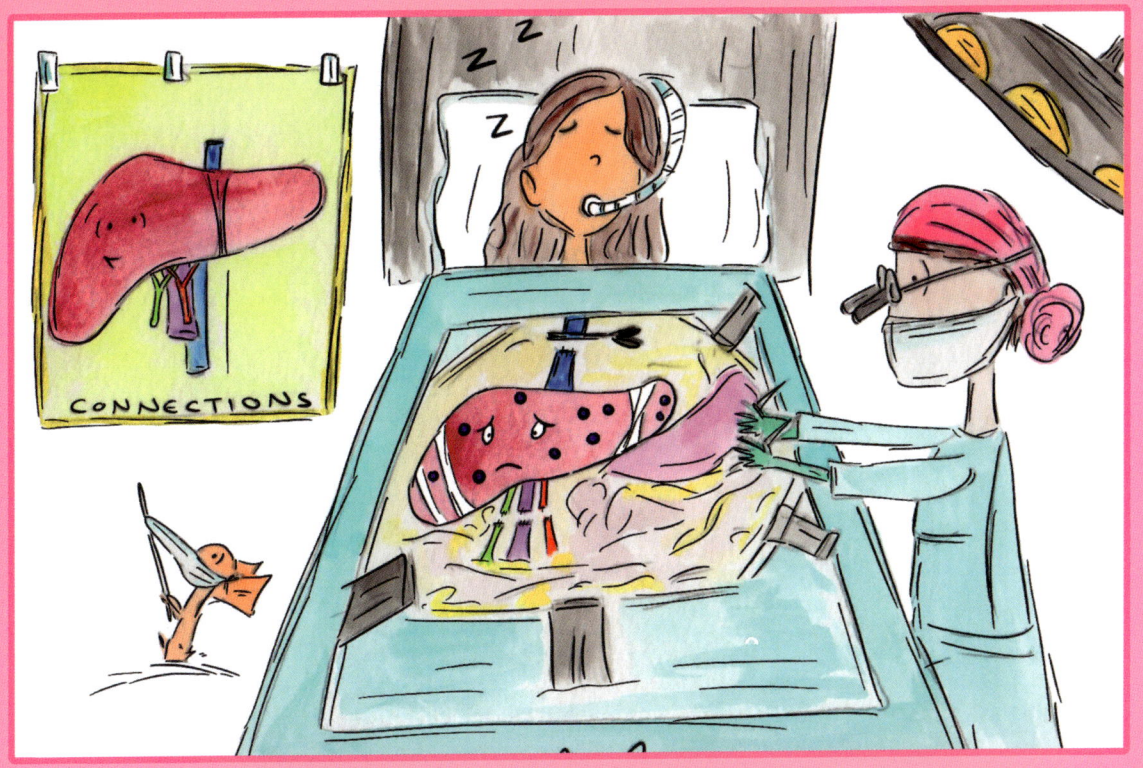

Step 4. The recipient hepatectomy

This is when your surgery starts! You will be taken to the operating room and put to sleep. Sweet dreams! While you sleep, your surgeons will be removing your sick liver. This is called the **recipient hepatectomy**. To remove it, it has to be disconnected from a bunch of pipes in your body. There are four pipes: the inferior vena cava (IVC), the portal vein, the hepatic artery, and the bile duct.

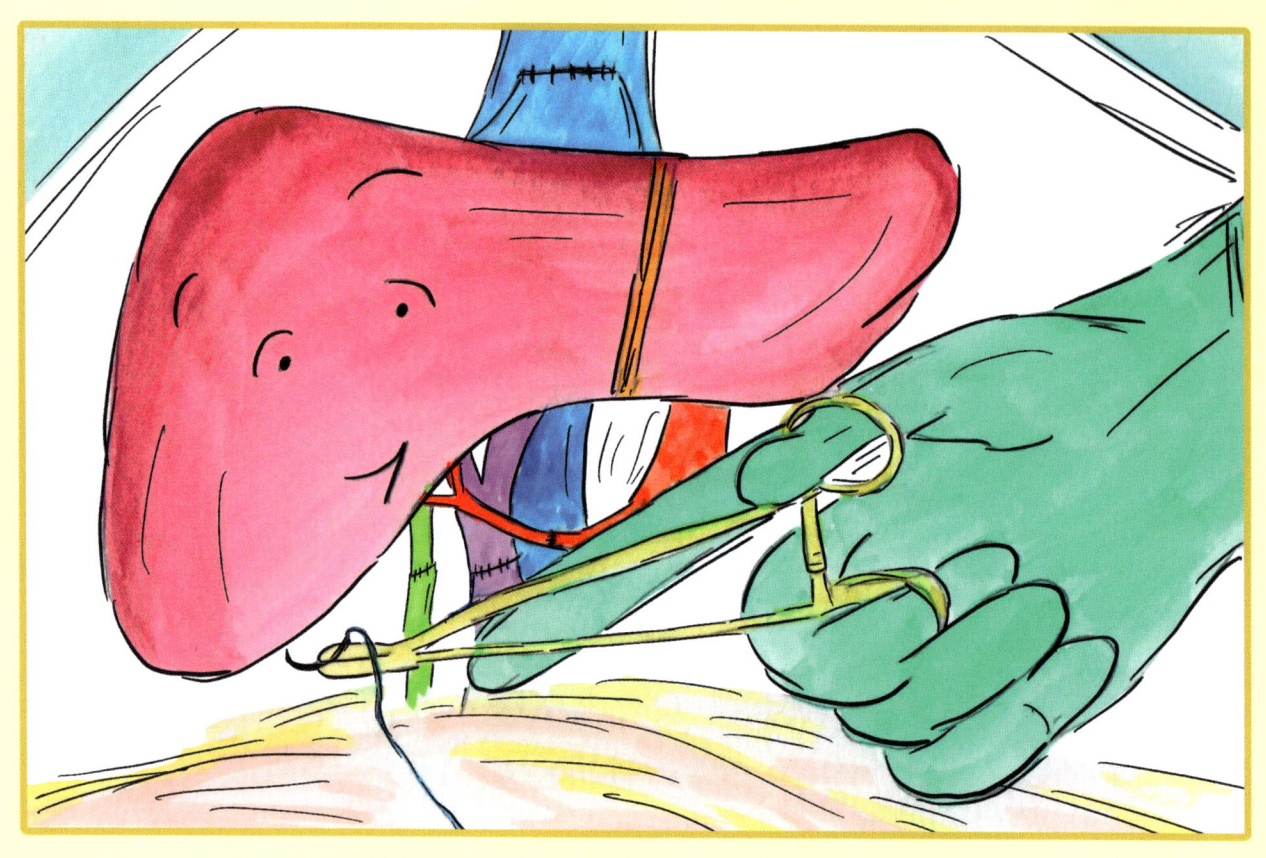

Step 5. Transplant time!

GO TIME! Let's put your new liver in. Your new liver – whether it's the whole liver, or a piece of a liver – needs to be connected to your four pipes. Your surgeons do that by sewing your new liver to them. Connection 1 – the IVC. Connection 2 – the portal vein. Connection 3 – the hepatic artery. And connection 4 – the bile duct! Your new liver is ready to rock and roll!

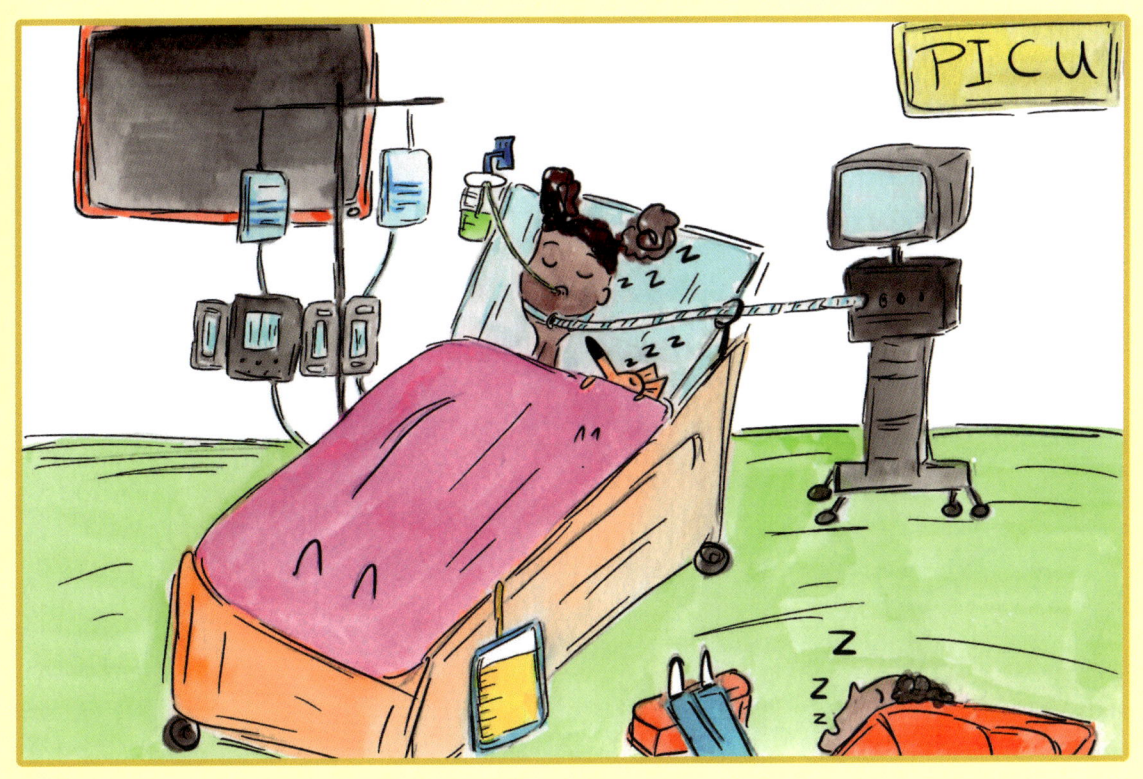

Step 6. Recovery

The first stop after surgery will be to the **PICU** – the pediatric intensive care unit. You will be sleepy and may have a breathing tube. Your nurses and doctors will keep a close eye on you and your new liver. They do this with **lab blood tests** and **ultrasounds** (a safe, painless way to take a picture of your liver using high-frequency sound waves). Check out all the tubes you may have and what they do on pages 18 & 19.

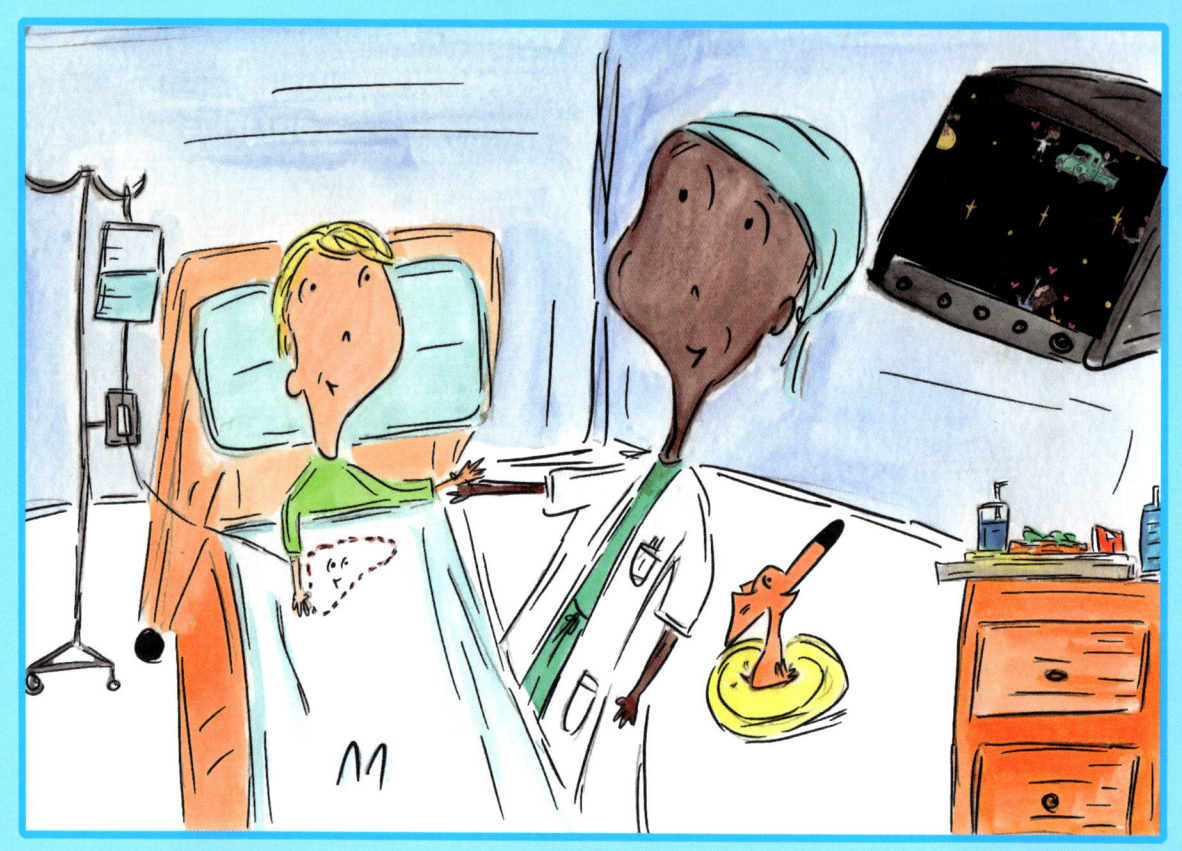

Step 7. Getting stronger

When your team thinks you're ready, you will be moved out of the PICU. This can be several days or longer. Your team will keep watching you for possible problems that can happen (see pages 20 & 21). In the meantime, you'll keep getting stronger. Take deep breaths, walk with the nurses, and eat good meals.

After several days, it may be time to go home!

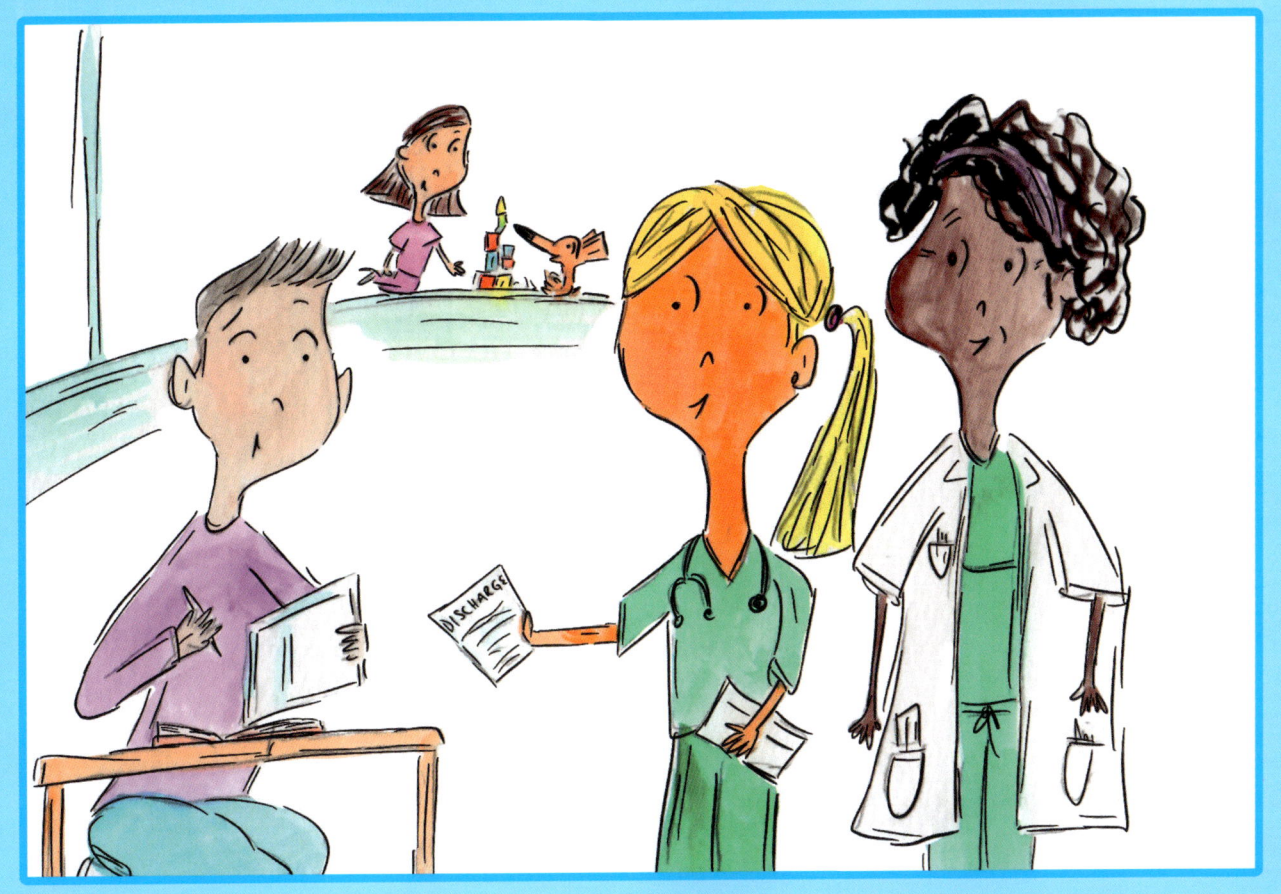

Step 8. Discharge

You and your parents will get all sorts of education. Education on your new medicines, your diet, your activity instructions. Education on caring for your new liver. Education on how to keep getting stronger! Every day you will feel better. And every day you will have more energy. Liver transplant is the best!

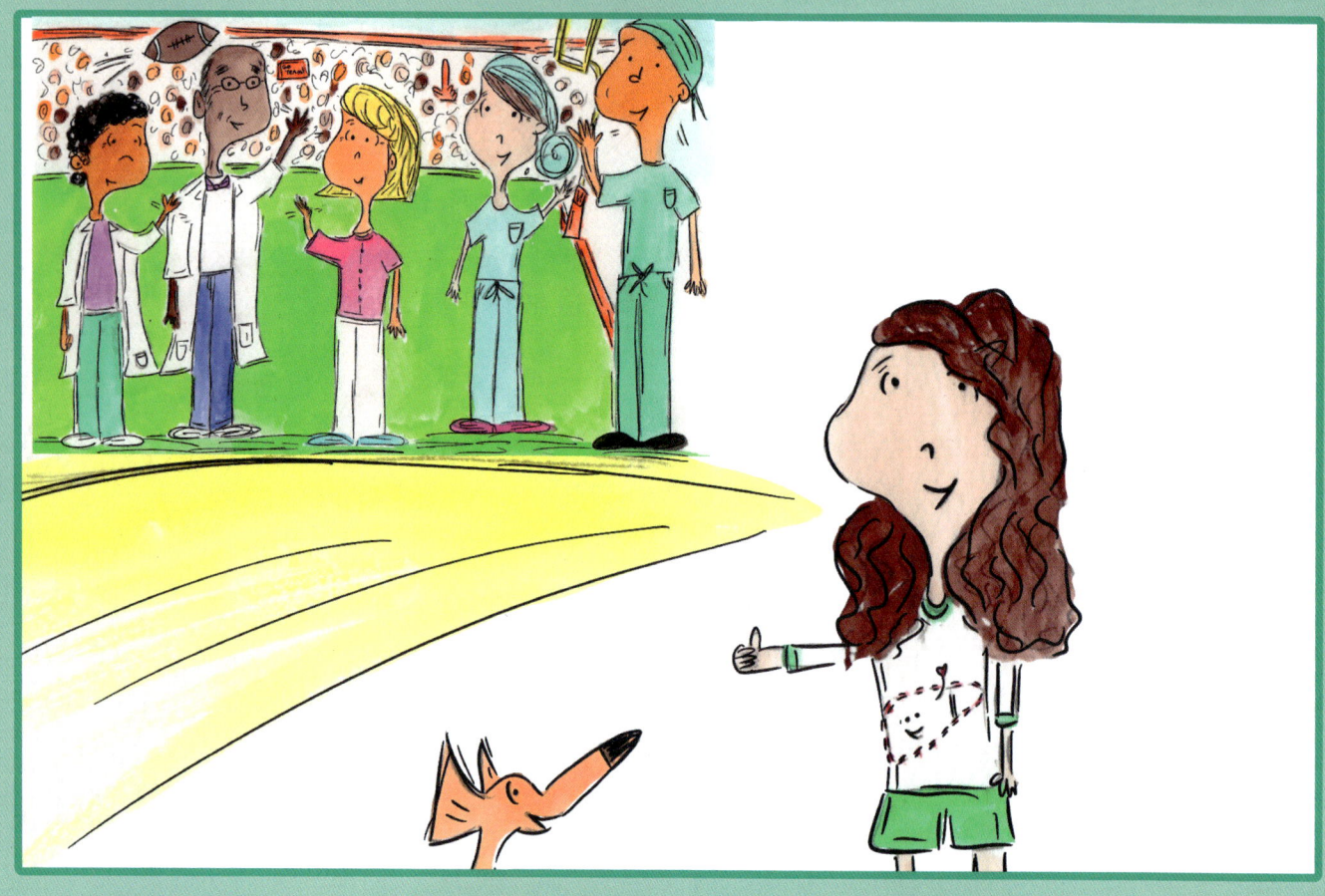

So, there you have it. You're all ready now for your liver transplant surgery when the times comes! And don't forget, you'll have a big team helping you and rooting you on every step of the way!

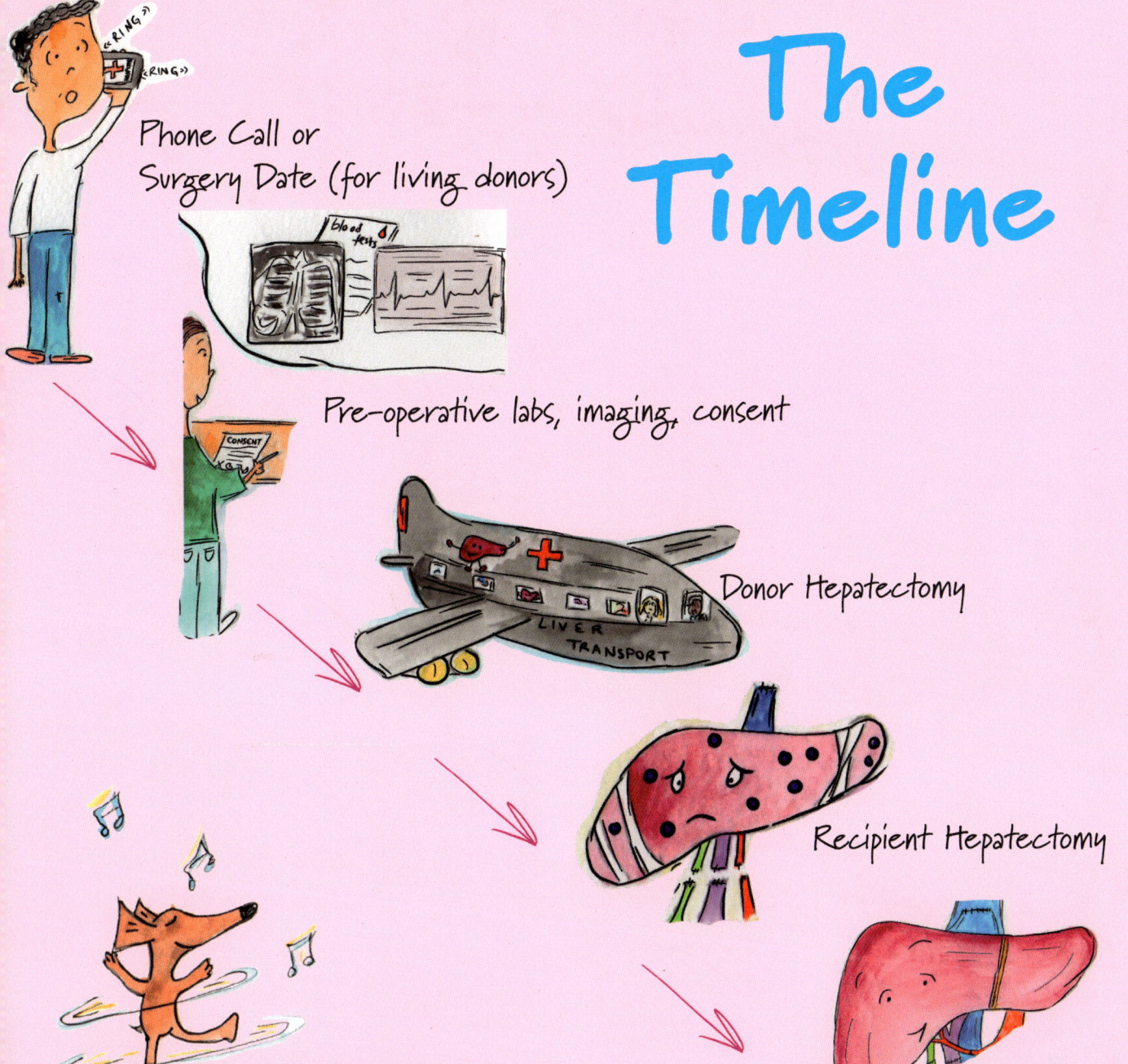

The Timeline

Phone Call or
Surgery Date (for living donors)

Pre-operative labs, imaging, consent

Donor Hepatectomy

Recipient Hepatectomy

TRANSPLANT 13

Surgery Details

So how long does the actual transplant surgery take?

Surgery time includes going to sleep, getting IV lines, placing a urinary catheter, getting you comfortable and secure on the bed, washing your belly, draping for surgery, and then the surgery itself! The actual surgery time itself depends on a whole lot of factors. For you, it will feel like a few minutes between going to sleep and waking up. For your family, it will feel like a few days because of worry and stress. And, just because a case goes longer than expected doesn't mean something is wrong. The operating room will call out to the waiting room with updates throughout the case. If there are problems, your surgeon will come out and speak with your family. Easier said than done but tell your family to try not to worry!

Now, in general, the transplant can take anywhere from 6 to 12 hours.

The surgery cut (incision) is usually an inverted 'Y'.

Once your sick liver is removed, the new liver has to be connected to your body. There are four connections that are made:

1) The inferior vena cava – this is the biggest vein in your body. It takes blood from your liver to your heart.
2) The portal vein – the portal vein brings blood from your intestines to your liver.
3) The hepatic artery – this is an artery that brings blood from your aorta (the biggest artery in your body) to the liver.

4) The **bile duct** – the tube that   drains the bile your liver makes into the intestines. This lets the bile break down fats in foods we eat.

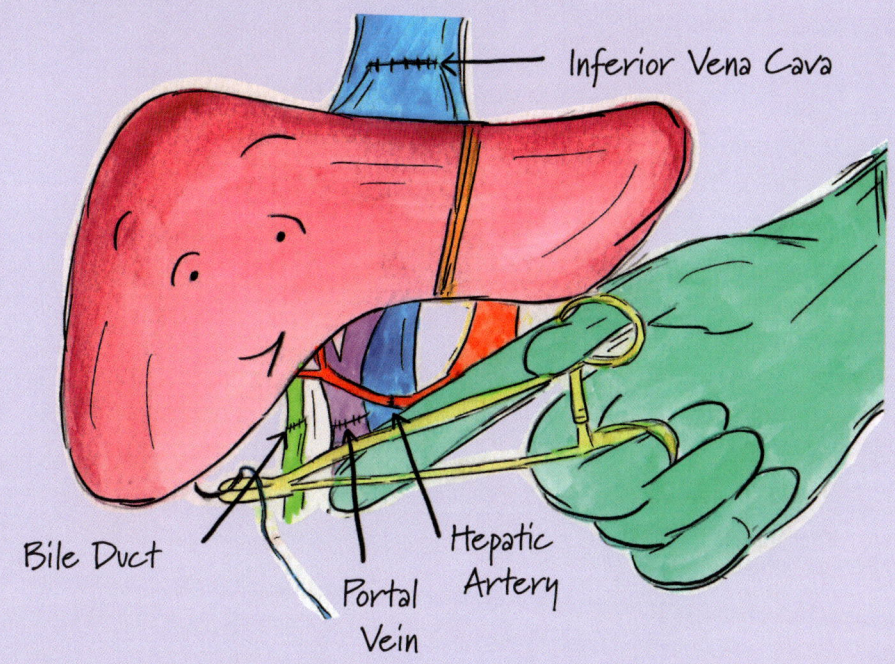

Inferior Vena Cava

Bile Duct

Portal
Vein

Hepatic
Artery

Your bile duct connection can be connected in one of two ways:

1) **Duct to duct** - this is when your old bile duct is sewn to your new transplant liver's bile duct (like the picture above).

2) **Roux-en-Y Hepaticojejunostomy** – this is when small intestine is connected to the bile duct.
We do this usually if you have a very small or very damaged bile duct. Or if you have no bile duct! Like in biliary atresia.

A drain will be left to drain extra fluid from your belly. This helps your surgery incision heal. The drain will be taken out usually before you go home.

What type of Liver did you get?

There are three different types of livers you may get!

1) **Deceased Donor Whole Graft** – This is when you get an entire liver from someone who no longer needs it.

2) **Deceased Donor Split Graft** – This is when you get a piece of a liver from someone who no longer needs it. We only take a piece so it fits your body!

3) **Living Donor Graft** – This is when someone alive (like your mom or dad or ever a stranger!) gifts you a piece of their liver!

The piece of liver (called the **graft**) that you get from a living donor or from a split liver depends on how big you are. The bigger you are, the more liver you need. The different possible pieces are:

- **The Right Lobe** – this is the biggest piece of liver so it's for big kids – like teenagers. It's the pink section below – made up of segments 5, 6, 7, and 8!
- **The Left Lobe** – this is the next biggest piece of liver so it's for children. It's the yellow section below – made up of segments 2, 3, and 4!
- **The Left Lateral Section** – this is the smallest piece of liver so it's for babies. It's a part of the left lobe - made up of segments 2 and 3 only!

16

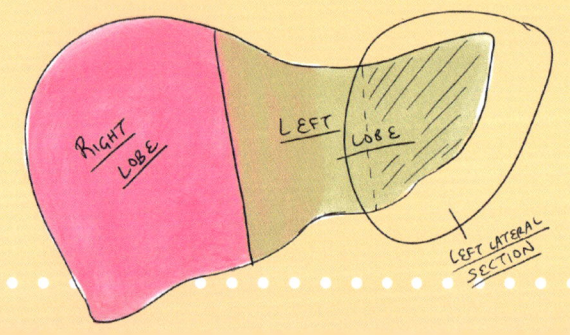

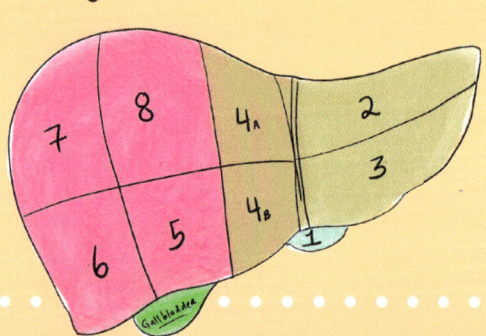

Watching your new Liver

Your transplant team will keep a close eye on you and your new liver after surgery. They do this with **lab blood tests** and **ultrasounds** (a safe, painless way to take a picture of your liver using high-frequency sound waves).

The ultrasound looks at the blood flow through your new liver. It looks at all your new connections! Sometimes, it may find a problem (like a clot).

Labs are drawn often after surgery. At least once a day. They look for lots of things. Some of those things are:

1) **Complete blood count** (called a 'CBC') – This includes your **hemoglobin** number which is often low after surgery from losing blood. Many patients need blood transfusions after surgery. It also includes your **white blood cell count** which lets us know if you may be getting an infection.

2) **Liver tests** – These labs include your **transaminases** and your **bilirubin**. They show how your liver is doing – if it is hurt or healing. After surgery, your liver tests might rise and fall like a rollercoaster! This is normal at first!

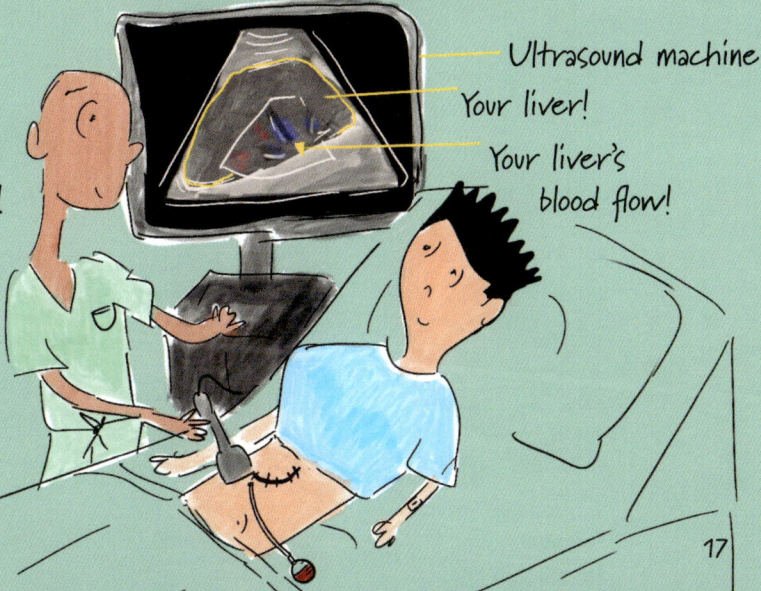

Ultrasound machine
Your liver!
Your liver's blood flow!

17

Tubes Galore!

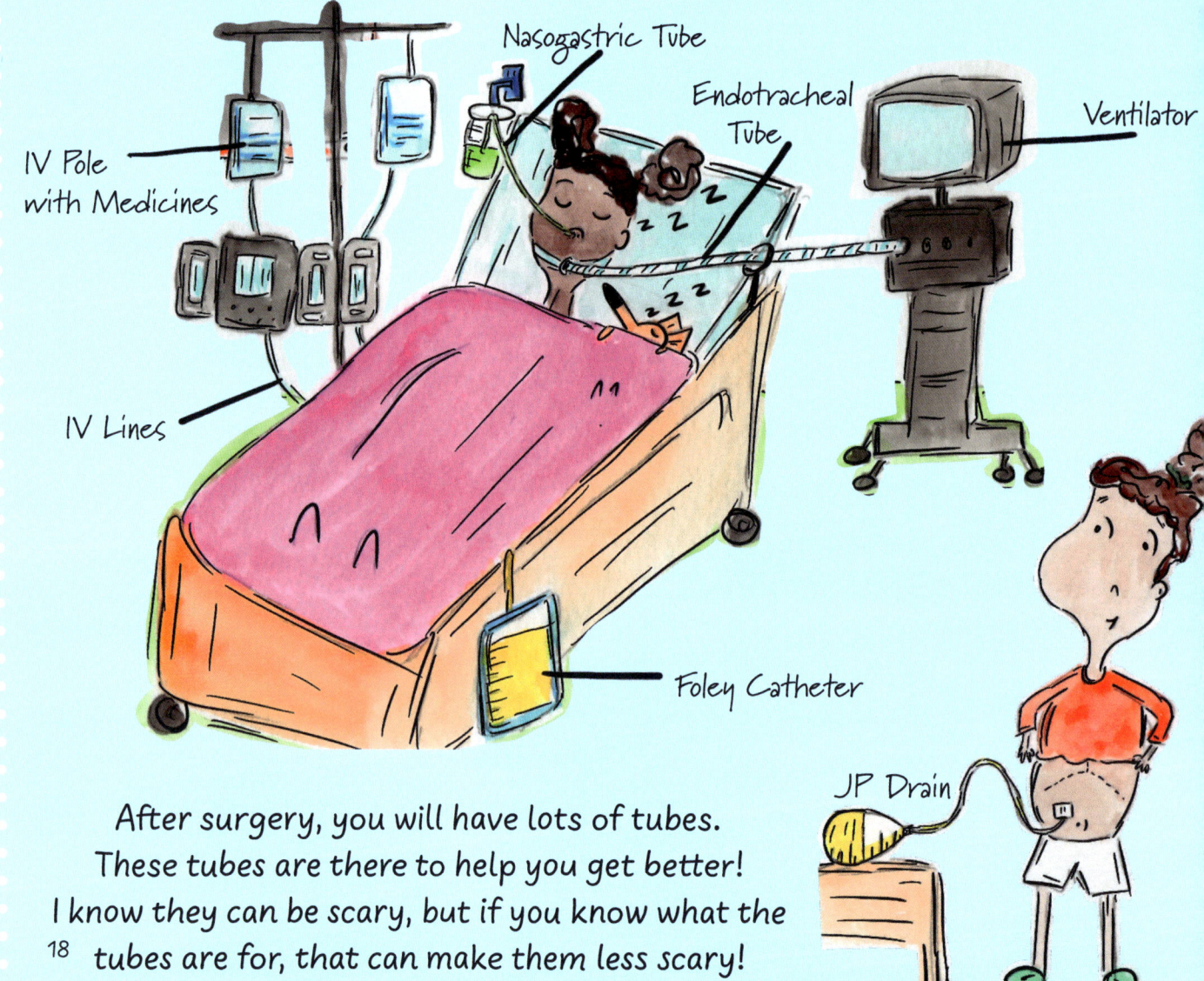

IV Pole
with Medicines

IV Lines

Nasogastric Tube

Endotracheal
Tube

Ventilator

Foley Catheter

JP Drain

After surgery, you will have lots of tubes.
These tubes are there to help you get better!
I know they can be scary, but if you know what the
tubes are for, that can make them less scary!

All these tubes will be removed at different times depending on how you are doing! Usually the first tube to go will be your endotracheal tube. And usually the last ones to go will be your IVs.

1. **Endotracheal tube** – this is your breathing tube! It is attached to a ventilator that breathes for you while you are sleeping. It is removed anywhere from hours to days after surgery.

2. **Nasogastric tube** – this tube goes from your nose into your stomach. It helps keep the stomach empty. If you have a roux-en-y bile duct connection, it usually won't be removed until you start farting or pooping. Otherwise, it may be removed earlier.

3. **IV lines** – you will have multiple IVs that will be used to watch your blood pressure and give you medicines.

4. **Foley catheter** – this tube goes into your bladder and collects your urine. It is usually removed a couple days after surgery.

5. **EKG leads** – these are stickers that are on your chest. They watch your heart rate and rhythm.

6. **Oxygen saturation probe** – this is a sticker that wraps around your finger or toe. It measures your oxygen level.

7. **JP drain** – this is a surgical drain. It collects fluid from around your liver while your body heals. You may have more than one. Usually, it is removed before you leave the hospital.

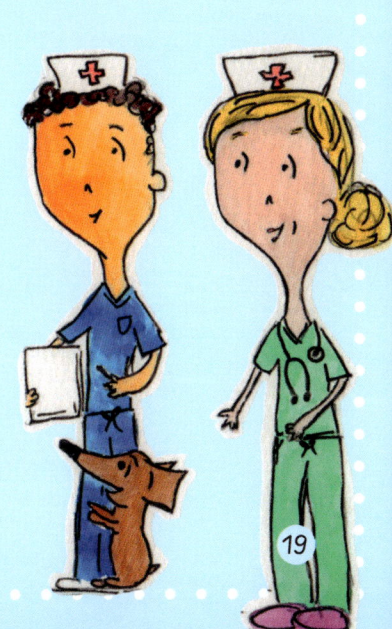

Possible Problems after Surgery

After surgery, your team will watch you closely for possible problems.
Most problems, if spotted early, can be treated!

Bleeding – This is common and is treated with blood transfusions. Sometimes, you may need another surgery to wash out the blood and stop the bleeding.

Primary graft non-function -This is super rare. It's when your new liver does not work. We don't know why this happens. If it happens, you'll need a new second transplant quickly.
– Signs – labs show your liver is not working
– Diagnosis – labs and liver biopsy
– Treatment – new transplant quickly!

Early allograft dysfunction – This is when your new liver doesn't work right away (within the first seven days after surgery). Over time, it can get better.
– Signs – labs show your liver is not working
– Diagnosis – labs and sometimes a liver biopsy
– Treatment – supportive care

Blood clots – The hepatic artery connection or the portal vein connection can get clogged by a blood clot (**thrombosis**).
– Signs – labs show your liver is not working
– Diagnosis – liver ultrasound shows the clot
– Treatment – Sometimes blood-thinning medicines, a radiology procedure, or a trip back to the opearting room to unclog it. You may even need a new transplant liver.

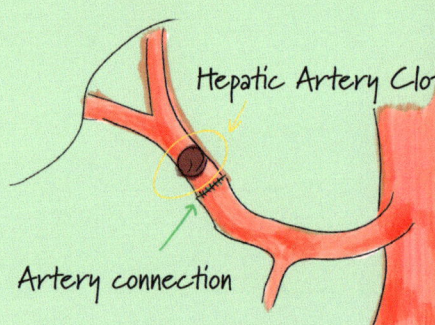

Hepatic Artery Clot

Artery connection

Bile duct complications – Sometimes the bile duct connection can leak or get blocked. Just like pipes under a sink get clogged.
– Signs – high liver enzyme labs, belly pain, fever
– Diagnosis – a painless x-ray (**cholangiogram**) to look at your bile duct
– Treatment – Depends on what we find. Might be medicines, cleaning
20   out the duct with an **ERCP** (defined on page 23), or very rarely surgery.

Biliary Stricture

Wound problems – Sometimes your surgery cut can have problems. That's why your team looks at your cut each time they see you. These problems can include infection, **hernia** (a hole in your belly wall, underneath your surgery cut), scarring, or **dehiscence** (when your surgery cut reopens).

Rejection- Your **immune system** is a part of your body that protects you from bad invaders – like bacteria and viruses. Since your new liver is a stranger to your body, sometimes your immune system will think it is actually a bad invader and attack it. It doesn't realize your new liver is there to help you! This is why it is important to take your medicines. Your medicines are called '**immunosuppression**' and calm your immune system down, so it won't hurt your new liver. You take these for the rest of your life because rejection can happen at any time.

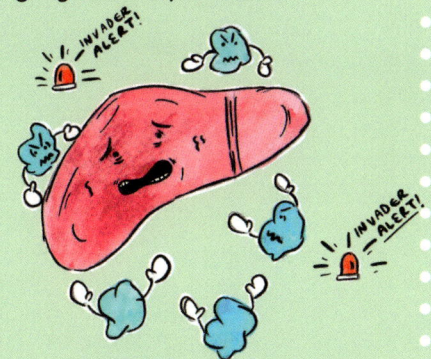

Immune System Cells

- **Acute rejection** is most common and is most likely to happen within 6 months of surgery.
- Signs – fever, decreased appetite, belly pain, high liver enzyme labs
- Diagnosis – liver biopsy
- Treatment – more immunosuppression medicines

Infection – Your '**immunosuppression**' medicines calm down your immune system, so it won't hurt your new liver. Unfortunately, this can slow down your immune system, so it's not as good at finding and destroying actual bad invaders – like bacteria or viruses that can cause infections. So, you'll take special medicines (like **antibiotics**) to help prevent infections from making you sick.

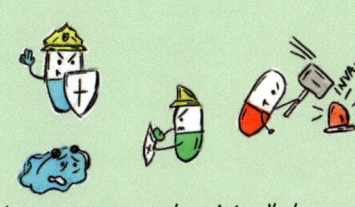

Immunosuppression Medicines

- Signs – fever, tiredness, diarrhea, throwing up, redness at your surgery cut, cough, sore throat
- Infections to watch out for -Thrush (oral yeast), respiratory viruses, CMV (cytomegalovirus), EBV (Epstein-barr virus), and Herpes

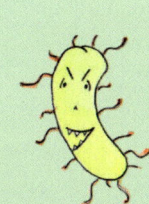

Staying up-to-date on your **vaccines** is also important and helps! Work with your liver team to know what vaccines you need and when!

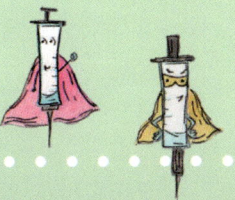

When to call your Team

Once home, call your team if you have any of the following:

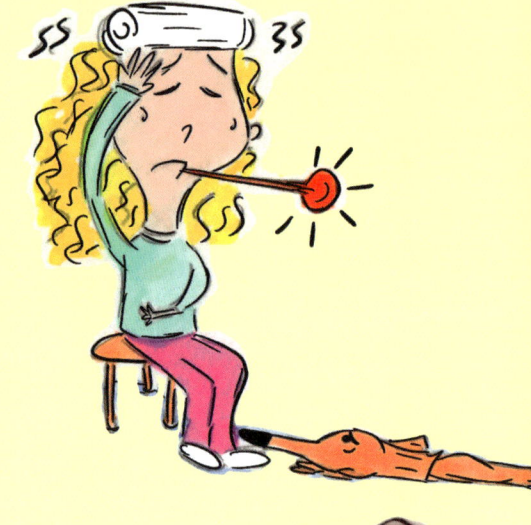

- Fever >100.5 degrees F
- Any flu-like symptoms
- Feeling sick to your stomach (nausea), throwing up, or diarrhea
- Belly cramps/aches
- Worsening pain or redness at your surgery cut
- Drainage at your surgery cut
- Pain when peeing or decrease in pee amount
- Change in your pee to cloudy, bloody or smelly
- Sore throat
- Feeling short of breath
- Having a cold
- Sores or blisters near your mouth
- Any and all questions!

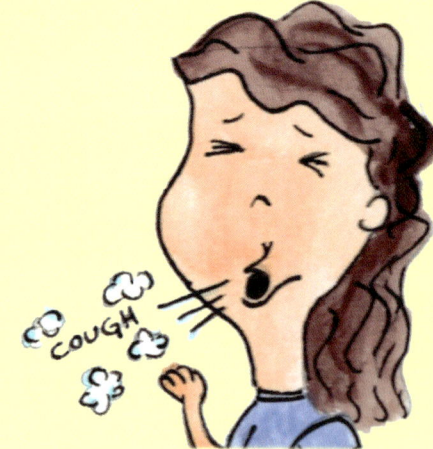

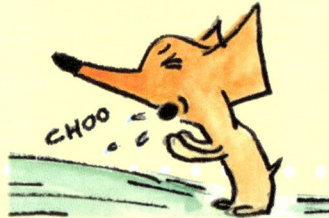

Doctor Words

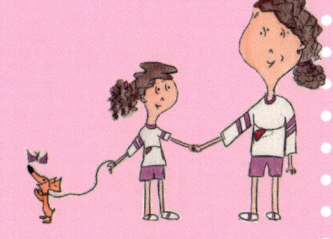

Living donor liver transplant – when you get a piece of a healthy liver to replace your sick liver from someone alive (like your mom or dad!).

Deceased (cadaveric) donor liver transplant – when you get a healthy liver from a person who has died and no longer needs it. If this liver is too big, we cut it into a smaller piece (**deceased SPLIT liver transplant**) so its fits in your body.

Recipient Hepatectomy – fancy words for the surgery to remove your sick liver.

Liver Biopsy – a small sample of your liver is taken with a needle when we are worried about problems after surgery like rejection. This is done by a radiology, hepatology, or surgery doctor while you are asleep, so you won't feel a thing.

Endoscopic Retrograde Cholangiopancreatography (ERCP) – a special procedure using a camera that goes down your mouth to help clean out or open your bile duct connection if it gets clogged. Don't worry – you'll be asleep during it!

Immune System – a group of cells in your body that protect you from infection. Sometimes it will attack your new liver which is why you take immunosuppression.

Immunosuppression – medicines to help slow down your immune system so it won't hurt your new liver. Unfortunately, they will also slow down and diminish your immune system, so it's not as good at catching bad invaders that cause infection.

Roux-en-Y Hepaticojejunostomy – when the bile duct connection is between your small intestine and the new liver's bile duct. We do this when you have a very small or very scarred bile duct.

23

Meet the Author:
Dr. Maria Baimas-George

Maria Baimas-George MD MPH is an abdominal transplant surgeon. Inspired by her patients and mentors, she writes and illustrates books explaining medical and surgical conditions to children and their loved ones. Her goal is to create books that provide useful information to help with understanding and to offer comfort and hope.

WINNER OF THE
2021 SILVER
TOUCHSTONE
AWARD

Awarded for exceptional performance in patient safety, clinical outcomes, efficiency & service excellence

Please visit us online at
www.StrengthOfMyScars.com to learn more about our team and story and see our full collection of available books.

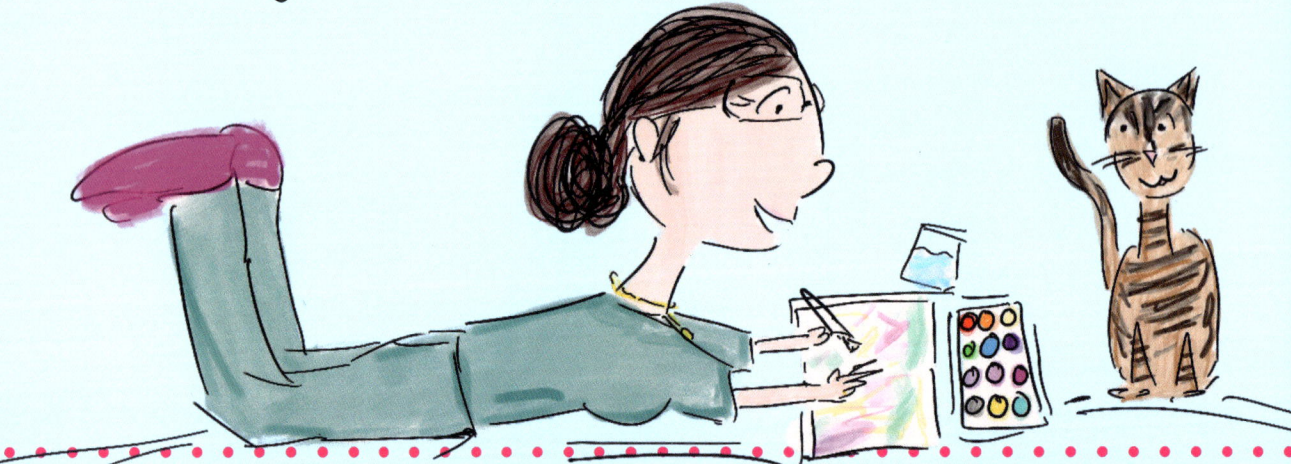